# Your Complete Keto Quick Start Guide: With 14-Day Diet Meal Plan and 42 Quick and Easy Recipes to Melt Away Stubborn Pounds Fast

Gretchen Freeman

# Table of Contents

# Introduction

Many suffer from various chronic conditions such as diabetes and obesity, and usually, the main culprit is the food they eat. The standard human diet contains high amounts of protein and carbohydrates, both of which are harmful to health because they end up provoking insulin and leptin resistance. As a result, you gain too much weight, contract inflammation, and develop the tendency to damage your cells. As such, significant food changes are needed, and the best way is to lead the body to a state of nutritional ketosis, a condition in which the body burns fat rather than sugar as a source of energy. To achieve nutritional ketosis, you must follow a ketogenic diet. But what exactly is a ketogenic diet?

The practice of the ketogenic diet has been in existence for almost a century ago. It rests on a solid knowledge of nutritional science and physiology. The ketogenic diet acts by targeting a host of underlying factors that are responsible for an increase in body weight, which includes abnormalities in hormonal regulations, especially the resistance of insulin, which contributes to increase in the level of sugar in the body. This factor is one of the benefits of the keto diet.

This keto quick start resource and guide will tell you everything you need to know about the ketogenic diet: how you can apply it to your lifestyle and what benefit you can get from it.

## Keto diet

A keto or ketogenic is a low carbohydrate eating plan that can help you burn fat more effectively. The typical ketogenic diet is a deficient carbohydrate diet. This was created for epileptic patients by researchers at the Johns Hopkins Medical Center. It was observed that fasting - by avoiding foods for a short time, including carbohydrates had beneficial effects on the number of seizures that patients experienced, and on the body's fat, cholesterol, and blood sugar. However, it is uncommon for people to go for long periods without food. The keto diet was, therefore, developed to produce results similar to fasting. Thus, it can be especially helpful in burning excess body fat without starvation.

For keto starters, the diet incites the body to act as if it is fasting (while obtaining the intermittent benefits of fasting), thanks to a reduction or removal of glucose in consumed meals. When foods containing carbohydrates are consumed, they are converted into sugar in the blood. If the blood sugar levels get too high, the extra calories will be stored as body fat, leading to an unwanted rise in body weight. On the other hand, when carbohydrate consumption is greatly reduced, the body begins to produce ketones from fat, and the level of these ketones in the blood can be measured using different methods.

Ketogenic diets, like some other diets, involve eliminating glucose. Since most people feed on high-carbohydrate diets, the body system has adapted to the use of glucose as our energy source. But once the supply of glucose to the body is limited, we start burning stored fat or the fat from food intake.

Therefore, when you follow a keto diet starter guide, your body burns fat and not carbohydrates to give you energy. This makes most people lose weight quickly, and their body fat excesses are rapidly broken down, even when they consume a lot of fat and enough calories daily. Another significant benefit of the ketogenic diet is that you don't need hours of strenuous physical activity to burn calories. As described above, when we eat very few foods that provide carbohydrates, we release less insulin. With lower insulin levels, the body does not store extra energy in the form of fat for later use, but can instead access existing fat stores for energy.

Keto diets are rich in healthy fats, and also tend to be very nutritious, which can help reduce the empty calories, sweets, and junk food that we consume. Many people have already experienced the many proven benefits for weight loss, health, and performance, as numerous studies show.

## Ketosis

"Keto", an abbreviation for the word ketogenic, is coined from the ability of the body to produce small fuel molecules called "ketones". Ketones are alternative sources of fuel for the body, which it uses when blood sugar (glucose) is low. Ketone production is usually a response to low carbohydrates level and moderate protein in the body system, which could otherwise be converted to blood sugar. Although dietary fats (especially saturated fats) often have a bad reputation, causing fear of weight gain and heart disease, they are also your body's second favorite source of energy when carbohydrates are not easily accessible.

The breaking down of fats into ketones takes place in the liver, serving as a source of energy for the entire body, especially the brain. The human expends a lot of energy daily, which makes it challenging to utilize fat directly as fuel, but can make use of glucose or ketones. When the body produces ketones, it goes into a metabolic state called ketosis. The fastest way to reach ketosis is through fasting, without eating anything, but this cannot last forever. Contrary to starvation, a keto diet can be followed for long periods, often leading to ketosis and weight loss.

A body is said to be in ketosis when the energy supply of the body comes majorly from ketones rather than glucose. This contrasts with glycolysis, where glucose is the major source of the body's energy. Therefore, ketosis is a condition in which the body burns fat rather than sugar as a source of energy.

## Keto-adaptation

For all of us in this fascinating world, I will tell you a little more about this concept: "keto-adaptation". There is a difference between keto-adaptation and ketosis. Many people experience ketosis when they sleep as their bodies are burning fat. However, this does not mean that your body is fully adapted to ketosis, for which your cells must develop new machinery and enzymes to burn fat.

Most people have been using glucose and sugar throughout their lives, and now we are adapting the body to ketosis, which is forcing our body to find different sources of fuel, and that can take around two to three weeks. Unfortunately, for some, it may take longer. Keto-adaptation is easier for some than for others.

When we start with a ketogenic diet, our body will first resort to stored glycogen, but this ends quickly (at first, we can feel a particular weakness). The process of obtaining energy through fatty acids and ketone bodies begins. In a balanced system, the muscles should get energy only from fatty acids and the brain only from the ketone bodies, but in reality, the muscles feed on both, and there is also a significant loss of ketone bodies through urine (which is why we test positive on ketone measurement strips).

Between two to three weeks, we should keto-adapt; that is, our body should be able to generate the ketone bodies exclusively necessary to feed the brain (we will lose that certain mental heaviness at the beginning). These ketone bodies will not be lost through the urine, and the muscles will be supplied exclusively with fatty acids (they have access to a practically unlimited supply of energy, which is particularly valuable for athletes). At this time, our test strips will stop marking positive, returning to the white color at the beginning of the process.

Some people experience changes in their body when they go from burning sugar to burning fat (these changes are known as "keto-flu"), or they may have rashes and all kinds of other body problems. They are all easy to handle, but, for many of those problems, you just need more minerals and B vitamins (nutritional yeast), sodium, or potassium. When you start consuming those nutrients, all these effects should be reduced. During this adaptation process, people begin to lose a little weight, but they will lose more afterward since they have not yet developed the full capacity of enzymes to burn fat. When you're fully keto-adapted, you could burn fat that you couldn't before.

**How do you know if you are keto-adapted?**
There are a couple of key signs. You don't have any more carbohydrate cravings, you are satisfied after eating, and your appetite is decreasing, especially between meals. Therefore, if you are not satisfied after eating while on the keto diet, it is because you still have an insulin problem, and you are not yet adapted. It can take about two weeks or even more to become keto-adapted.

Other signs of being keto-adapted are the following:

- you do not have headaches

- you do not have high blood sugar

- you are not in a bad mood if you skip a meal

- your mood is much better

- you do not have keto-flu

- no feeling of tiredness

4

- stability

- satisfaction

- you do not need snacks

- you can go long periods without eating


If you experience all or some of these changes, let us tell you that you are already keto-adapted. In summary, Keto-adaptation is the process by which the human body metabolism adapts to using ketones optimally as an energy source, getting used to doing it continuously in periods of carbohydrate shortages.


## Fat-adaptation

"Fat-adaptation" and "keto-adaptation" are two similar metabolic states, however, with subtle but meaningful nuances. That said, you follow some steps to get to both.

Fat-adaptation refers to a metabolic state in which the body burns fat for energy. Fat-adaptation involves training the body to burn fat — rather than glucose — for fuel. You can become fat-adapted without being in ketosis and vice versa. You don't have to adhere to a keto diet to reach fat adaptation. You can eat vegan, primal, or paleo diets or observe fasting to stay in this state — but you are not in ketosis. You are not in ketosis if your body is not producing ketone bodies to use for energy. However, you can remain in a fat-adapted state through other means, such as fat oxidation. Also, to become fat-adapted, eating a low-carb, high-fat diet and aiming for a carb intake between 20-50 grams per day will help your transition from burning glucose (being a sugar burner) to burning fat stores (being a fat burner).

When you start the keto diet, and you vastly reduce your carb intake, your body quickly burns off all remaining carbs and glycogen stores. Then, when carbs are no longer available, it begins to utilize excess fat reserves for energy. After about four weeks or more, your body becomes "fat-adapted". In this state, you've almost lost your cravings for carbs; you eat less and still feel great. Also, once fat-adapted, consuming food having a little higher carb intake in a day won't affect your ketone and blood glucose levels as much as it would while you were transitioning from a high-carb diet.

It generally takes from 30 days - 12 weeks of eating ketogenic diets without cheats or deviations to become fat-adapted. During this period, you'll experience two different phases. The initial phase, carb withdrawal, lasts for about three to 14 days and is characterized by cravings, hunger, and maybe the keto flu. The second phase follows suit, where your body is adjusting from relying on glucose for energy to relying on fat, which can last six to eight weeks. After several weeks, your body is on fat-burning autopilot, and that's where you'll stay as long as you maintain a keto lifestyle.

To become fat-adapted, gradually reduce the consumption of foods high in both carbs and sugar, replacing them with high-quality proteins and healthy fats. However, if there is any need for you to consume carbs at all, consume foods with a high amount of dietary fiber. Eat healthy fats from coconut oil, avocados, and olive oil, and high-quality protein from grass-fed meat, seafood, and eggs.

The word "slowly" should be emphasized, that is, going from eating 100 grams of carbs to 10 grams overnight is not easy on your body. Rather than cut carbs out entirely, which can cause adverse effects including nausea, headaches, brain fog, and other symptoms of keto flu, it is advisable to ease the transition slowly and steadily.

Reduce carbs little by little, simultaneously adding in more healthy fats and protein to ensure you're consuming enough calories.


## Who should not keto diet?
While the keto diet has many proven benefits, it is, however, not without some controversies. Generally, it is considered safe for most people. The list below composes of the groups of people who are advised not to keto diet:

| Class of people | Reasons |
|---|---|
| Pregnant women | A pregnant woman needs nutrients v various sources. Therefore, severe deprivation of healthy carbohydrate sources could adversely affect the baby's health. |
| Lactating women | Women should avoid the ketogenic diet throughout the breastfeeding phase. This is because a keto dieter limits the intake of oxaloacetic acid, an essential substance for producing lactose for breast milk, which is necessary for the growth of babies. |
| Athletes who are about to start a new season | Athletes can benefit significantly from the energy produced by ketones, but it takes about four to six weeks to reach ketosis. During this time, the body is still not used to using fat as a source of energy, which can worsen your performance in upcoming athletic competitions. If you want to get the benefits of a ketogenic diet, give your body time to adapt by planning it during the break between one season and another. |

| | |
|---|---|
| People who have had their gallbladder removed | The gallbladder collects and contains bile, allowing the digestive tract to absorb dietary fat properly. Without it, dietary fats will not be completely absorbed, which can lead to nutrient deficiencies, as a ketogenic diet relies heavily on nutrient fats. The solution is quite simple. Make sure you take two supplements (ox bile and lipase) for every meal that contains fat. Ox bile will help you to emulsify fats to absorb them, acting like the bile released by the gallbladder. Lipase is an enzyme that will help you digest fat. |
| People who suffered from kidney stones | If you have had experience with kidney stones in the past, a ketogenic diet could increase the chances of them coming back. This is because ketones are naturally acidic, and increase the production of uric acid and the formation of stones. On the other hand, kidney stones can be avoided during a ketogenic diet by increasing potassium consumption through green leafy vegetables and other fatty foods, such as avocados. Keeping hydrated throughout the day also helps reduce the risk of stones. |

| People who are still growing | In a study, epileptic children who were given a ketogenic diet showed reduced symptoms and improved cognitive performance. However, according to a publication in the Journal of Developmental Medicine & Child Neurology, consuming a keto diet can hurt the growth of their bodies in the long run. The researchers argue that the ketogenic diet reduces the production of insulin-like growth factor type I (IGF-1), a hormone essential in the development of the bones and muscles of children and adolescents. If your child necessarily needs a ketogenic diet, you must first consult a doctor to discuss potential growth problems. |
|---|---|
| Skinny people by nature | Anyone skinny by nature, and has a body mass index (BMI) of less than or equal to 20, should avoid the ketogenic diet because it could lead to further weight loss, dangerous for their general health. |

| | |
|---|---|
| Those with rare metabolic diseases | Disorders such as Gaucher disease, Tay Sachs disease, Niemann-Pick disease, and Fabry disease can interfere with fat metabolism, thereby affecting energy production. If you have one of the ailments above, a ketogenic diet is not recommended, since it relies heavily on energy-producing fats. |
| Anorexics | Anorexics who follow a ketogenic diet run the risk of suffering hunger quickly because their calorie consumption is already limited, and they have an extreme fear of eating fat, abundant in this diet. If they undertake a ketogenic food plan, they may suffer from low energy, because fats are the primary source of energy. However, with the support of medical care and psychiatric supervision, their overall health could benefit from ketones. |
| Pancreatic insufficiency | In this disorder, the pancreas fails to produce enough enzymes to help break down and absorb nutrients in the digestive tract. If you have an enzyme deficiency, I would suggest treating it before starting the ketogenic diet; otherwise, the gastrointestinal tract would have difficulty absorbing dietary fats. |

**Health benefits**

Keto diets are rich in healthy fats, and also tend to be very nutritious, which can help reduce the empty calories, sweets, and junk food that we consume. There are a lot of stories from people who have followed a keto diet to improve their health. The benefits are similar to those of other low-carb diets, but appear to be more potent than low-carb diets. Look at the keto diet as a super-loaded, low-carb diet that maximizes benefits. These benefits include:

- **Weight loss**

Keto diet decreases your insulin levels considerably and increases your ability to burn fat significantly. This makes it easier for you to lose body fat without hunger.

- **Control of appetite**

A keto diet gives you new control over your appetite. When your body burns fat, it has constant access to weeks or months of stored energy, significantly reducing the feeling of hunger. Studies have shown that this ability to control your appetite is a common experience, making it more comfortable to eat less and lose excess weight; you just need to wait until you're hungry to eat. Many keto dieters eat twice daily, even once for some other people. Not having to fight hunger can also help with problems like sugar or food addiction, and possibly with eating disorders like bulimia. At least feeling satisfied can be part of the solution. Food can stop being your enemy and become your friend, or just feed you, as you prefer.

- **Reduce the risk of heart disease**

Both triglycerides and high cholesterol are known markers of diseases associated with the heart. The keto diet most probably doesn't harm the level of your cholesterol, even though it includes a lot of fat. Besides, it acts by lowering these risk factors as found in people with obesity. For example, it was found that those who followed ketogenic diets for 24 weeks had lower triglyceride, LDL (Low-Density Lipoprotein) cholesterol, and blood glucose levels among many patients while HDL (High-Density Lipoprotein) cholesterol level increased.

- **Control blood sugar and reverse type-2-diabetes**

The ketogenic diet helps control blood sugar levels. It is also excellent for controlling type-2-diabetes, and sometimes even leads to a complete reversal of the disease. This has been proven in various studies. It makes perfect sense since the keto diet reduces the need for medications, lowers blood sugar levels, and reduces the potentially negative impact of high insulin levels. Since a keto diet can even reverse existing type-2-diabetes, it is likely to be effective in preventing or reversing pre-diabetes.

- **Energy and mental performance**

Some people follow ketogenic diets specifically to increase mental performance. Also, it is common for people to experience an increase in energy when they are in ketosis. The brain of a keto dieter feeds on ketones 24-hours, 7-days a week, and ketones are efficient fuel for the brain. Thus, ketosis produces a constant flow of fuel (ketones) to the brain, avoiding the problems experienced with massive changes in blood sugar. Sometimes this could translate into improved focus and concentration and resolution of mental haze or clouding, with improved mental clarity.

- **Increased physical endurance**

In theory, keto diets can increase physical endurance by improving access to large amounts of energy in fat stores. Unlike the body's glycogen that only lasts for a couple of hours of intense exercise or less, fat stores carry enough energy to last for weeks. Another potential benefit is the reduction in the percentage of body fat that can be achieved with a keto diet. This decrease in body fat weight is potentially valuable in several competitive sports, including endurance sports.

- **Fight against brain diseases and neurological disorders**

Keto diets have played important roles in the treatment and reversal of cognitive impairments and neurological disorders such as Alzheimer's symptoms, epilepsy, anxiety, and manic depression. Research shows that depriving the body of glucose through diets that are very low in carbohydrates allows the body to produce ketones as fuel. This helps the reversal of cognitive impairments and neurological disorders, including inducing the control of seizure. This alternative energy source can be used in place of the faulty energy pathways in brain disorder patients.

The keto diet helps to normalize the symptoms of pathophysiological processes in schizophrenic patients such as delusions, lack of control, hallucinations, and other behaviors. Also, it helps to reverse the side effect resulting from the use of medicines for treating brain disorders, such as weight gain, cardiovascular risks, and type-2-diabetes.

- **Longevity**

Some evidence suggests that diets that are low in carbohydrates (such as ketogenic diets) extend life span in contrast to low-fat diets. The Lancet, a medical journal, carried out a study on over a hundred thousand adults in 18 countries and associated high carb intake with a high mortality rate. In contrast, each fat type and total fat intake were associated with lower overall mortality. The fats were not associated with mortality from myocardial infarction or any other cardiovascular disease.

The study also presented a reduced risk of having a stroke, that is, the more a person consumes saturated fat daily, the more they appear to be protected from a stroke attack. The ketogenic diet also induces autophagy, removing damaged and senescent cells from the body. The induction of autophagy is a bio-hacking technique to help eliminate the signs of poor aging, and keto dieting is one way to achieve it.

The above benefits are the most common. Also, a keto diet can help control migraines.

# Plan your diet

The diet to lose weight rapidly is low in carbohydrates. The ketogenic meal plan restricts you to consume as few carbohydrates as possible. Your gender, age, activity level, and body composition helps to determine your carbohydrate and fat intake. Your food should be primarily high in fat and moderate in protein because protein excesses are converted into blood sugar in the body. Avoid low-fat diet products. A rough guide is about 5% carbohydrate (the fewer the carbs, the more effective the diet), 15-25% protein, and about 75% fat.

The rules below can guide you through keto dieting:

- **Adequate protein intake but don't load protein.**

The protein content in keto diets differentiates it from other low-carb diets. Protein is not as important as fat in a keto diet. In small quantities, the body breaks proteins into glucose, which indicates that if you overeat, especially at the beginning, it will delay your body's transition to ketosis. Your protein consumption should be between 1 and 1½ g/kg (0.001 and 0.0015 lb/lb) body weight. Divide your ideal weight by 2⅕ to change pounds (lbs) to kilograms (kg). For example, a woman weighing 72 kg (150 lbs) should consume about 72 to 108 g of protein per day.

- **Combine your diets with supplements**

Popular keto supplements can help you get results faster and stay that way. Blackberry ketones are not exogenous ketones, and so you don't have to use them since they do not increase ketone levels in the body. Also, the amino acid, leucine, should be supplemented since it can be converted to acetyl-CoA in the body. While other body amino acids help glucose formation, the acetyl-CoA formed is helpful to produce ketones. Also, it is present in foods such as cottage cheese and eggs.

Medium chain triglyceride (MCT) oil is another essential supplement that is most commonly extracted from coconut oil. It is often added to bulletproof coffee, salad dressings, keto shakes, and herbal teas. As the name implies, this type of oil contains medium-length chains of fats called triglycerides. Due to its shorter length, MCTs are easily digested and converted to fuel (ketones) almost immediately after ingestion. MCT oil offers many significant benefits, aside from weight loss. These include blood sugar control, helping the body go into ketosis to use body fat for energy, acting as a source of energy that can also be used to fuel the brain, and control of epilepsy, Alzheimer's disease, and autism.

- **Drink water**

Water is essential to life. Having enough water is vital for digestion, detoxification, and reduction of tiredness and hunger. Try to drink about 11 cups of water daily.

- **Limit carbohydrate intake**

Do not consume above 20 g of carbs per day (fiber exclusive). The less the sugars, the more effective the keto will be.

- **Avoid snacking**

When you feel like taking snacks, ask yourself if you are starving or not. If you have eaten enough with meals, you will no longer need to snack.

- **Don't cheat**

Finally, cheating is not allowed on the keto diet, because eating food with too many carbohydrates will get you out of ketosis. In fact, if you cheat, expect some symptoms of keto flu to show up, but if you had been in ketosis before, returning to ketosis will be sooner and faster than initially.

## Types of keto diets

The traditional keto diet, created for people with epilepsy, was to absorb about 75% of the calories from fat sources (such as oils or fatty pieces of meat), 5% carbohydrates, and 20% proteins. The macronutrient percentages in this ketogenic meal plan for epileptic patients are strict. For most people, a lighter version (what I call a "modified keto diet") can still help promote weight loss safely and often very quickly, but we have many other types of ketogenic diets.

Here are the most common types of ketogenic diets:

- Standard keto diet: about 75% of the calories are from fat sources, about 20% of the calories are proteins, while the remaining 5% are carbohydrates.

- Modified keto diet: here, the meal plan limits calories to 30% carbohydrates while the protein and fat compose of about 30% and 40%, respectively.

- Cyclical keto diet: this option is your bet if you have trouble sticking to a very low-carb diet for months. Carbohydrate cycling only increases your carb intake with the right amount when appropriate, usually about once or twice a week.

- Targeted keto diet: this keto diet plan permits you to add carbohydrates during exercise only. So, you will eat carbs on workout days.

- Restricted keto diet: some studies have shown that calorie restriction and ketosis can help in cancer treatment, so this meal plan limit calories and carbohydrates.

- High protein keto diet: this is common among people who want to maintain muscle mass, such as bodybuilders and the elderly. Protein forms about 30% of the calories, with 65% fat, and about 5% carbohydrates. (Please note: people with kidney problems should not increase their protein intake).

- Vegetarian diet: this menu contains many vegan foods rich in carbohydrates and nutrients. Low-carb nuts, seeds, fruits and vegetables, leafy vegetables, fermented foods, and healthy fats are excellent choices for this plant-based diet.

- Dirty keto diet: the percentage of carbohydrates, protein, and fat are similar to that of a standard keto diet, but here, you can eat lots of naughty fats instead of the healthy ones. This is not recommended.

- Lazy ketogenic diet: finally, this diet is often confused with dirty keto, but they are different because the term "lazy" means not carefully following the calories or macros of protein and fat. Although lazy, this diet does not allow you to eat more than 20 grams of net carbohydrates daily. A lot of people find this diet less intimidating, but you may also not be impressed with your result.

Before putting together a practical list of foods for the ketogenic diet, it is initially essential to take a look at what you eat and get rid of all that is unhealthy. You must eliminate sugars, starches, packaged, and processed foods from your diet because the ketogenic diet is based on real foods.

**What can you eat?**

Concerning specific foods to include in a ketogenic diet, as well as those to eliminate, here is an overview of what you could choose from a grocery store:

- Vegetables: when setting the food plan of a ketogenic diet, it is essential to focus on green leafy vegetables because of their fiber, antioxidants, and different nutrients. The best ones include broccoli, spinach, parsley, Brussels sprouts, courgettes, mushrooms, tomatoes, carrots, broccoli, cabbage, spinach, kale, sea vegetables, peppers, etc. Some should help you keep your carbohydrates clean to a minimum.

- Fruits: although fruits are generally healthy, in a ketogenic diet, you should avoid most of it because they are real natural sweets with high amounts of sugar. However, following a diet low in carbohydrates and high in fat like the ketogenic diet does not rule out eating all fruits. But, in principle, you can't eat most fruits on a keto diet. And the sweetest fruits are usually the tastiest, such as peaches and melons. However, you don't have to exclude all fruits in the keto diet. Here are some fruits that can be eaten in moderation without breaking your ketosis: avocado, tomato, blackberry, raspberry, strawberry, olives, lemon, and coconut. For other fruits, unfortunately, they are too rich in carbohydrates to be eaten whole.

- Healthy foods that are low in sugars or carbohydrate-free but high in protein: these include bone broth, grass-fed meat, cage-free eggs, wild-caught fish, pasture-raised poultry, organ meats, dairy products, raw goat, cheese, olive oil, palm oil, nuts, coconut oil, seeds, and grass-fed butter.

**What can you drink?**

As for drinks, you have several choices. The most important is water, but you could also drink organic black coffee (without sweeteners or milk), which is rich in antioxidants. You can also drink coconut milk and herbal tea because they contain many antioxidants and nutrients.

**What should you avoid?**

- Carbohydrates: carbohydrates (carbs) that contain a lot of sugar and starch. These foods are very high in carbohydrates. Basically, on a keto diet, you have to avoid sugary foods altogether, as well as starchy foods like bread, pasta, rice, and potatoes.

- Avoid processed and ultra-processed foods: these foods have high calories but low nutrients. These include products with white or wheat flour, bread, conventional dairy products, and other processed grains such as pasta, boxes of cereals, sweet snacks and sugary drinks, and pizza.

- Milk: avoid drinking milk, because it contains galactose carbohydrate. Drinking just one glass can make you reach the expected amount of carbs for a whole day. Also, avoiding dairy helps people who have lactose intolerance to take on the ketogenic diet.

- Also, many other products should be avoided, such as hydrogenated vegetable oils (canola oil), soy-based foods, and carbonated drinks. They may contain few carbohydrates, but they are unhealthy and can destroy your health.

# How to start
# the keto diet

The actual ratio of recommended macronutrients (or "macros") in your daily diet can vary. Historically, a targeted keto diet has been to limit carbohydrate intake to 20 to 30 grams net per day. "Net carbohydrates" are the number of carbohydrates remaining after the dietary fiber is considered. Since fiber is indigestible when consumed, most people do not include grams of fiber in their daily carbohydrate allowance.

**total carbohydrates - grams of fiber = net carbohydrates**

In a standard keto diet, fats generally provide between 70% and 80% of total daily calories, proteins between 15% and 20%, and carbohydrates barely 5%.

## Guide to start the ketogenic diet

Here's what the ketogenic diet offers. We increase our consumption of fat, which will become our primary source of energy, and we reduce carbohydrates to 20 g/day. Protein consumption remains moderate. By respecting the ration of 75% good fat, 20% protein, and 5% carbohydrate, your liver will produce ketone bodies, which is to say energy made from lipids (fat) and only after a few days of carbohydrate reduction. But in the first few weeks, the ketones will be released into the breath and the urine. You will have a funny breath or smell, similar to nail polish. This is because our cells have always used glucose (energy produced from glucose) as an energy source, so it takes a period of adaptation. It can take up to four weeks before your mitochondria (the energy factories in your cells) use ketones as an energy source. We then say that you are keto-adapted. Your breath and urine will return to normal.

You will also notice that you are less hungry, and the cravings will disappear. After a few months, your blood tests will improve (may take up to six months), and your physical condition will improve. You are going to lose weight and have more energy. Ketones are the ideal fuel for our cells, including our heart and brain cells. Indeed, the combustion of ketones in the mitochondria is 25% more efficient than the burning of carbohydrates. You will feel less pain. Unlike glucose, ketones do not excite the brain since they stimulate the production of GABA (a brain inhibitor, a natural calming type). This is the reason why ketones soothe pain and have a general anti-inflammatory effect.

During the adaptation period, you may experience specific side effects, such as the keto cold, that is, you will have the impression of having a cold. These are simply manifestations of carbohydrate withdrawal that lasts an average of a day or two. It is vital during this period to increase your salt intake (1 teaspoon sea salt in a glass of water, up to two per day). You are no longer eating processed food; you are now eating a more natural diet, so you are consuming less sodium.

Depriving the body of carbohydrates will also lower the level of insulin in the blood and reduce the level of water and sodium stored in the kidneys. Your sodium and electrolyte levels will be lower. This drop in electrolytes can also cause leg cramps at night.

During adaptation periods, it is essential to drink lots of water, increase your salt intake, and consume broths of chicken or beef bones. You may also need to add magnesium and potassium, especially if you have leg cramps at night.

But to start, I recommend that you only cut the carbohydrates - limit yourself to 20 g per day. For the protein serving, eat a source of protein with each meal. One serving is the size of the palm of your hand and the thickness of a deck of cards. Add fat to each meal, such as fatty meat, avocado, oil, homemade mayonnaise, butter, etc. If you eat enough fat, you shouldn't be hungry until the next meal. If not, increase your fat. We must not limit calories; we must feed our fill. You don't count calories; that's another myth since cutting calories doesn't lose weight. Just start to tame this new way of eating. When you are comfortable, you can start counting your macronutrients.

**Quick start guide**

Starting a new diet plan does not have to feel intimidating but should instead be exciting, especially if you have taken steps to deal with any obstacles to come. When starting the keto diet, for example, you may feel different effects during the initial stages, including some that are unpleasant. Eventually, the payoff of the keto diet is usually worth it; just keep in mind that some patience might be required. This would probably be a moderate or significant change for the average person's diet. You have to reduce your carb-based food intake, which means minimizing everything from grains to even most fruits and increasing your meat and healthy fat intake.

If you have decided to try the keto diet plan, this guide will explain what you can expect for the four weeks and beyond, as well as offer tips to help you respond well. Take before and after photos and a record of weights for each week of the keto diet.

## Week 1

Firstly, remember that any keto side effects or challenges you might experience are temporary and usually harmless. It is common to start losing weight in as little as early as three days, which can be highly motivating for the dieter diet. However, this depends on how well you adhere to the keto diet plan. If you restrict your daily carb intake below 20 grams, it takes about three days to go into ketosis. The loss of weight in the first week is mainly due to water loss. If you have a little water to lose, it may take a few weeks to start seeing real weight loss and vice versa.

When you are starting the ketogenic diet plan, you are much more likely to be successful if you work according to a plan. Prepare for the keto diet by planning your meal, grocery shopping, and cleaning out your kitchen. (follow our 14-day meal plan and pantry list for grocery shopping).

Since most people are accustomed to using carbs/sugar for energy, it takes a few days of starting a keto diet to enter ketosis. When your carb intake drops below around 50 g a day, your body enters a state of ketosis; your cells switch from burning glycogen (energy from carbohydrates) for fuel to burning ketones that result from fat metabolism. This is a significant change for your body to undergo.

Therefore, the first five to seven days on a keto diet can feel a lot like having the flu called keto flu. Unlike most common flu, it is not contagious, but it can be unpleasant. Keto flu symptoms do not affect everybody but are common. These symptoms most likely occur during the first five to seven days of the menu plan, usually between one to two weeks, although it might take some until three to four weeks to recover fully. These include fatigue, constipation, increased food cravings (especially for sugar and carbs), headaches, muscle weakness, insomnia, moodiness, brain fog, and lack of concentration.

At the start of the keto diet, the first day always feels great because you still have some glycogen to burn. However, after about two to three days, physical and mental fogginess begins to set in, often with staring at the wall for extended periods, feeling half-drunk, and being unproductive at work—the primary reason being that your brain is used to burning glycogen for fuel. As a result of the change in the form of energy supply to your neurons, your cognitive function will start to decline. However, the cloudiness generally clears after a couple of days, and you will experience an elevated sense of mental clarity when your brain starts burning more ketones for fuel (usually after one or two weeks).

To alleviate this physical and mental fogginess: go super low on carb for the first week (consuming less than 10 g of net carbs daily). This forces your body to use up your glycogen stores and get into ketosis much more quickly. Also, consuming MCTs when you start to feel fatigued is helpful. MCTs are the only fats that are transported directly to the liver, where they are broken down into ketones. Using this fatty acid supplement will provide your brain with more fuel, so it does not struggle when your glucose levels are low. Eat more low carb vegetables - the potassium, manganese, and iron content of green vegetables all play a crucial role in maintaining consistent energy levels and keeping your mind clear.

For difficulty in sleeping, you need to get enough sleep since a decrease in carbs affects your sleep patterns. Practice good sleep hygiene – it is not a good idea to exercise too close to bedtime. Reduce unnecessary noise pollution in your house or bedroom. Prioritize sleep and stress-relieving activities.

Besides, this transition to keto diets may also result in frequent urination caused by the breaking down of glycogen in your muscles and liver. This leads to dehydration or low level of electrolytes like sodium and potassium in the body. To mitigate these keto symptoms, stay hydrated by drinking enough water. Ensure you drink at least two liters of water a day, and if you are still thirsty, drink more. Tea and unsweetened coffee are allowed but stick to one or two cups. Stay away from alcohol, except for small amounts of organic red wine or low-carb beer occasionally. Try to replenish those lost electrolytes by eating plenty of potassium-

and magnesium-rich foods such as avocado, tomato sauce, spinach, salmon, and nuts. Adding extra salt to your food is enough to supply the body with sodium. Since you will be eliminating many foods from your diet, there is a chance you might experience a nutrient deficiency or require more specific vitamins and minerals. It is a good idea for most adults on the keto diet to take a daily multivitamin, an omega-3 fish oil supplement, probiotics and a magnesium supplement. These help to fight inflammation, constipation, low energy, and poor digestion. Also, adding exogenous ketone supplements (such as a ketone salt that contains Beta-hydroxybutyrate) to your routine helps to boost your body's ketone supply, which can help you get into ketosis more quickly and stay there.

At the end of the first week, you will likely see a significant drop in weight. Regular exercise, coupled with a typical menu with a caloric deficit, can make most people lose 1-2 lbs within a week. In contrast, those following a keto diet typically see a drop of anywhere 2-10 lbs. Implement these relevant strategies, and you will be able to alleviate the keto flu symptoms and other body changes that you may experience during the first week of keto dieting.

## Week 2

Take your pictures, recheck your weight and waist circumference. The second week of the keto diet is considered a continuation of the transition phase - in which your body is undergoing significant metabolic changes, leading to the adaptation phase. The symptoms of keto flu are expected to continue in the second week in some people. But many people find that after initial symptoms subside, the keto diet gives them more mental clarity, helps them feel more energized and healthier, and diminishes their sugar and carb cravings.

Many people often lose between 2-8 lbs within two weeks of following a ketogenic diet without cheating. But since our body differs from one another, some other factors may influence the way the body responds to keto diets. These factors include genes, gender, age, physical activity, etc. So, you don't have to blame the diet or yourself if you are yet to lose weight. Stick to the diet, and you will certainly lose those extra pounds, but it may take you extended periods compared to some other people because your body is still adjusting to its new source of fuel.

Reflect over the last two weeks and note any other improvements. Sluggishness usually set in during week 2. If this is the case, your diet is working — your body is switching from one energy source to another, and you will get your results soon. If symptoms persist, stay hydrated by drinking enough water as dehydration is often the culprit. It is an excellent time to start adding electrolytes to your diet since ketosis pulls water out of your cells. Take in plenty of salt and electrolytes. Also, withdrawal from junk and processed foods for your keto diet means you might not be getting the sodium you're used to, therefore add high mineral sea salt to your diet to prevent cramps and dehydration.

Sleep deprivation makes the keto flu worse, so make sure you're getting enough sleep as possible. Many people feel more energetic, lighter and even start to see some weight loss at the end of week 2. Hang in there if you're not one of them. Your reward will come soon, so don't be discouraged. Remember, breaking a habit of high carb consumption doesn't come easy, and it could get uncomfortable as your body reacts both mentally and physically.

**Week 3**

Take your pictures, recheck your weight and waist circumference. Week 3 is an adaptation phase. Depending on how strict you've been, your body should have either switched over (adapted) or be on the verge of switching over to burning fat. Consider testing your ketone levels with ketone strips or any other methods to ascertain if you're in ketosis. If you're not, continue with your meal plan, and you should get into ketosis soon.

By the end of week three, the keto flu symptoms should have abated. If side effects persist, that is, if you still feel crummy, review the principles of your diet and make sure you're following it correctly. A breakdown of your calorie intake should be as follows: about 75 % high-quality fats, 20 % protein, and only about 5–10 % carbohydrates. It is expected that by the third week, you should be more comfortable with what you can eat, and you might start looking for substitutions for your favorite foods. Failure to consume enough fat, eating too many carbs, or overeating protein will prevent you from experiencing real benefits and staying in ketosis. If you experience lots of hunger, likely, you could be dehydrated, or you are not consuming enough healthy fats or calories or. Track your macros to be sure you're on the right track.

You should carefully monitor your net carbohydrate intake during this phase to help your body adapt. To maintain ketosis, it is

24

advisable to keep your carb intake below 20 g per day. Cheating can be detrimental or even counterproductive while the body is trying to adapt to the changes in metabolism and diet, and might lead to weight regain and also give rise to cravings. If you are maintaining a deficit in your calories, you will start losing some fat. So, to achieve a stable and constant loss of weight, watching your calories is essential, which will be much more comfortable as a result of reduced hunger levels.

Your caloric deficit determines the weight loss you can expect, which can be about 1-2 lbs for the 3$^{rd}$ week onwards or even more. Lean people might struggle to lose the last few pounds, while weight loss in those that have more fat in their body will be more rapid. Many people would have begun losing weight by week 3, and many report increased energy to think clearly and more in-depth, but if you haven't, don't get discouraged; it will come soon.

## Week 4 and beyond

Four to five weeks into the diet, the early side effects of the diet will be gone. If you're sticking to the diet correctly, and not cheating, your body will actively be burning fat for energy. Congratulation, you are now fat-adapted!!! Since your body has now adapted to using fat as its main source of fuel, you will observe improved strength and endurance. The side effects experienced in the previous weeks should have entirely subsided. You might observe no craving for carbs, improved workouts, and sound sleep.

You can now be less strict with your net carbohydrate intake. You can experiment to know your limit (each person's carb tolerance is dependent on their body metabolism and level of activity). At this stage, although you still have to take caution and track your macros, you might feel better consuming a little bit over 20 g of net carbohydrate daily. Some people can consume about 30-35 g per daily and still maintain ketosis. Based on your goal and body, you may increase your carb intake once weekly or monthly, when you become fat-adapted.

Maintaining a constant weight loss of about 1-2 lbs every week depends on your activity level and caloric deficit. Women experience fluctuations in the amount of weight loss, which can be a result of their menstrual cycle, and people with very little weight to lose do struggle a lot more. Keto supplements like MCT oils provide more energy to the body, enhance weight loss, and are even helpful to overcome plateaus. If you engage in exercises regularly, your muscle weight will increase, such that it affects reading on the scale. If you are in ketosis and you are not losing weight, cut some calories. Focus on the big picture, which is: eat high-fat diets, keep protein moderate, and keep carbs low to keep yourself full.

The monthly average weight loss on keto is about 4-10 lbs (1-2 lbs a week, which is considered safe). Purchase and use a scale that measures the fat percentage in your body as another guide along your journey. Taking pictures is another great way to see changes in your body that may not reflect on the scale.

The weight loss result varies wildly and is a factor of how long and how well you stick to the diet plan. If you follow the keto diet appropriately, you should see a loss of at least 1 lb of fat for week 4 onwards. In 90 days of a continuous keto diet, you will likely see some significant weight loss results. Those who have substantial weight to lose could drop as much as 30 lbs of fat by this time. After three months, it gets even more challenging to get rid of those final pounds to reach your targeted weight. Stick to the keto diet, and you will see those last pounds ease off eventually.

## Quick 14-day diet start plan

Studies have shown that those following a keto diet typically consume below 50 g of carbs and approximately 1.5 g/kg body weight of protein daily. To stick to our macronutrient ratios of 75% fat, 20% protein, and 5% carbohydrate, we need to plan our meals. Here is a start 14-day diet meal plan:

The provided nutritional value represents the net carb.

| Day | Breakfast | Lunch | Dinner |
|---|---|---|---|
| 1 | Scrambled eggs<br><br>1 g | Keto cauliflower mac and cheese<br><br>3 g | Keto carbonara<br><br>2 g |
| 2 | Spinach and feta omelet<br><br>5 g | Tuna with vegetables<br><br>2 g | Shrimp avocado cucumber salad<br><br>5 g |
| 3 | Dairy-free latte<br><br>1 g | Keto caprese omelet<br><br>4 g | Pesto chicken and veggies<br><br>5 g |
| 4 | Keto fatty coffee<br><br>0 g | Caesar keto salad<br><br>4 g | Salmon with walnut-avocado guacamole<br><br>2 g |
| 5 | Avocado and pepper omelet<br><br>3 g | Keto shrimp & artichoke plate<br><br>7 g | Zoodles with creamy salmon sauce<br><br>9 g |
| 6 | Keto porridge of coconut and blueberries<br><br>7 g | Smoked salmon-filled avocados<br><br>7 g | Spicy kimchi ahi poke<br><br>3 g |
| 7 | Rolled smoked salmon, cream cheese and cucumber<br><br>2 g | Keto salami salad<br><br>2 g | Ketogenic pizza<br><br>5 g |

| | | | |
|---|---|---|---|
| 8 | Raspberry chia seed pudding<br><br>4 g | Spinach and bacon salad<br><br>3 g | Keto fried chicken and broccoli<br><br>5 g |
| 9 | Peanut butter yogurt and cocoa powder<br><br>5 g | Keto BLT sandwich<br><br>2 g | Eggs with salmon and spinach<br><br>2 g |
| 10 | Keto pancake<br><br>3 g | Keto Italian plate<br><br>8 g | Cabbage and bacon keto<br><br>7g |
| 11 | Chocolate chia pudding<br><br>6 g | Keto crustless pizza<br><br>5 g | Keto apple Dijon pork chops<br><br>2 g |
| 12 | Keto sandwich<br><br>4 g | Chicken no-noodle soup<br><br>4 g | Mexican cauliflower rice skillet<br><br>5 g |
| 13 | Keto zucchini hash<br><br>4 g | Keto frittata with avocado and queso<br><br>4 g | Salmon with asparagus & quick blender hollandaise<br><br>3 g |
| 14 | Mushroom omelet<br><br>5 g | Keto smoked mackerel salad<br><br>4 g | Oven baked trout with mustard glaze<br><br>8 g |

## How to measure ketone levels

If your goal is to take full advantage of the benefits of ketosis, we recommend that you measure your ketone levels more accurately to ensure that you are experiencing the benefits that we already mentioned. There are three ketone bodies: acetoacetate, beta-hydroxybutyrate (BHB), and acetone. As ketosis progresses and its concentration increases in the body, ketones can be detected in breath, blood, and urine.

## Detection of ketones in urine

The use of strips is the most comfortable and cheapest way to know if you have an adequate level of ketones in the body. Ketosis measuring strips are accessible, and you can find them in pharmacies, supermarkets and also online. There are different brands: Ketostix® and Keto-Diastix®. This method helps to determine the concentration of acetoacetate in the urine. The urine strips are also straightforward to use since once immersed in urine, they will begin to change color, and depending on how dark or light they are, you can have an approximate amount of ketones present.

The major demerit of this method is that the level of ketones in urine can be modified. Some factors raise the concentration of ketones in urine, while some decrease the concentration of ketones in the urine. The level of ketones in urine increases at the start of a keto diet or during the adaptation period, dehydration, fasting, and exercise. Meanwhile, ketone concentration decreases in urine during a high degree of hydration, after eating, and when you adapt to the keto diet.

## How to use the strips to measure ketones in urine?

Now that you know some of the situations that can alter the result of urine ketones, if you decide that they are the option you want to use, we recommend that you follow the following steps. You should use the strips, preferably every day at the same time, and remember to wash your hands before and after using them. To use this method, you will need to urinate into a container and immerse the strip in the sample for a few seconds until you notice a color change. Once the color changes, you can find out the concentration of ketones in your urine. The thickness of the color is proportional to the concentration of ketone.

The color chart printed on the packaging allows you to compare the color and therefore determine the approximate amount of ketones present in the urine. An approximate value between 15-30 mg/dl (1.5-3 mmol/l) can be targeted for optimal ketosis.

## Detection of ketones in the blood

With this test, you mainly measure beta-hydroxybutyrate (BHB), and it is the safest and most accurate way of knowing the concentration of ketones in your body. After three to five days of starting the keto diet, the body enters slight ketosis with values of 0.5-1.0 mmol/L. It takes a few weeks to reach the optimal level of ketones in the blood that is 1.5-3.0 mmol/L. Once this level is reached, you can be sure that your muscles and brain will receive enough energy from fat. Despite being the most accurate way to know ketosis, it has some disadvantages that you should know: it is more expensive, and it is also a more invasive method.

## How to measure ketosis in blood?

A glucometer-like device is used (you're probably familiar with it if you know someone with diabetes). This device is a reader that can measure the concentration of ketones with a single drop of blood from your finger. To use it, follow the next steps, remembering to wash your hands before and after. With a lancet, you must prick your finger to obtain a drop of blood, and then you will place it in the indicated place on the strip. Insert the strip into the reader. In a few seconds, you can know precisely the concentration of ketones, and thus you can be sure when you are at the desired value of 1.5-3.0 mmol/L.

## Detection of ketones in breath

This method is the least invasive, cheapest, but also the least non-specific method. It makes use of a device that you can also buy online, and it mainly detects acetone. The method of measuring ketones in the urine is useful, especially during the early weeks of starting a keto diet. If you have been months and these levels in urine "normalize," the strips may stop being a good option. If you do not want to prick your finger to know the level of ketones in the blood, then the measurement of ketones in breath can be an excellent option for you.

It involves the use of an installed program on your computer or a downloaded application on your phone. Once installed, you just have to breathe in the indicated place for 10-20 seconds and see the color code or the value to know the level of ketones in your breath.

## Which method is appropriate for me?

Once you know about the keto diet and ketosis in the body, you may understand the importance of accurately measuring the number of ketone bodies in your body. The most important thing here is to choose the method to measure these ketone bodies so that you are sure that you are achieving the benefits of this diet.

First, you must determine if you are willing to prick your finger to use the blood measurement method. It is not very painful, but it is something that many of us would prefer not to deal with day by day. If, on the contrary, it does not bother you, then you have found your perfect method. In case it is not an option for you, you could use the urine measurement method for the first month, and once you stop noticing the result in the urine strips, it means that you are in the adaptation phase. There you can choose the breath test. We remind you that ketosis measurement could be a great tool to ensure that the benefits of the keto diet are already taking effect.

## When is the right time to take the test?

The most appropriate time to take the measurements is in the early evening (in the morning upon rising, the amount of ketones in the urine is generally low). Otherwise, during the day, choose a time when you have already spent your physical activity but which does not immediately follow an intense effort. Different studies indicate that the longer you are in ketosis, the more beneficial the ketogenic diet is. However, it is not recommended to exceed 80 mg/dl (dark purple). If this happens to you, increase your carbohydrate intake slightly and ask yourself if you have had enough fluids. If you significantly exceed this level, this may be an indication that your body is having trouble with the metabolism of ketones. This situation is scarce, but it requires immediate medical attention from your doctor.

## Track your progress

Tracking your diet is highly recommended since you are new to the menu. It's easy to go over your carb limit or to miss your protein targets. You can get a smartphone app explicitly designed for the keto diet. Not only will you find hundreds of keto-friendly recipes, but you will also be able to plan and track your food quickly.

It is essential to track your macros - your grams of fat, protein, and net carbohydrates (not to be confused with calculating calories). Tracking your macros and carbs can be difficult, so I recommend downloading a keto app that includes a keto diet calculator such as a keto diet app and a keto tracker. These apps will help you achieve weight loss by keeping you on track.

# Possible side effects of keto diets

Changing your body's metabolism from burning carbohydrates (glucose) to burning fats and ketones at a sudden can have some side effects as your body gets used to its new fuel, especially after two to five days. Symptoms can include headache, tiredness, muscle fatigue, cramps, and heart palpitations. These side effects are often short-lived, and there are ways to minimize or cure them. Another option to reduce possible side effects is to decrease your carbohydrate intake gradually over several weeks. But with a slower start, you may not see spectacular results or feel the benefits so strongly.

Therefore, it is recommended that you leave sugar and starches in one go. You are likely to lose several pounds in a few days. While much of the rapid weight loss at first is water weight (decreases bloating), it's still a very motivating and inspiring way to start your keto journey.

The side effects of a ketogenic diet include the following:

• Keto flu

Most starters of the keto diet experience some symptoms of the keto flu. You may feel this, more or less, a few days after starting a keto diet. These symptoms include headache, fatigue, dizziness, light nausea, difficulty concentrating (clouding), lack of motivation, and irritability. These symptoms usually disappear within a week, as your body adjusts to the increased ability to burn fat.

The leading cause of keto flu is that carbohydrate-rich foods can cause water retention (bloating) in the body. When you start a low carb diet, much of this excess fluid is lost. You may notice an increased need to urinate, and with that, some extra salt is lost, resulting in dehydration and a lack of salt before your body adjusts. This is the main reason behind most keto flu symptoms. These symptoms can be decreased by consuming enough water and salt. Ensure you drink a cup of broth, one to two times a day.

- Short term fatigue

At the beginning of a ketogenic diet, you may begin to feel tired. It is one of the main reasons why many decide not to continue with this approach for a long time, even before enjoying its benefits. The reason you initially feel so fatigued is that the body is adapting to the use of healthy fats as an energy source rather than carbohydrates. The transition does not happen overnight, and the body could go into ketosis at any time from seven to thirty days.

- Bad breath

Once you start a ketogenic diet, you may notice that your breath smells terrible due to the increase in acetone levels in the body. Acetone is a ketone produced during ketosis, excreted through the urine, and partly through the breath. On the positive side, detecting acetone in your breath is an excellent indicator that the ketogenic diet is working. To try to eliminate the bad smell, you can brush your teeth or rinse your mouth with coconut oil.

- Frequent urination

During the first few days of the ketogenic diet, you may notice that you go to the bathroom more often. This is because the body is discharging the liver and muscle glycogen in the form of urine. And when insulin levels in the blood begin to drop, excess sodium is excreted in the urine.

- Digestive problems

A massive change in any diet can increase the risk of digestive issues, and the ketogenic diet is no exception. Constipation is commonly reported by those who start it, but it could disappear in a couple of weeks, as soon as the body gets used to the healthiest food you eat.

- Sugar cravings

When the body switches from using sugars to using fats, you may have extreme sugar cravings. However, I advise you not to fall into temptation. You can try some relaxation techniques such as the emotional release technique or yoga to distract you from the urge.

- Hair loss

During the first few days of the ketogenic diet, you may begin to find more hair attached to the brush. Don't panic, because hair loss can manifest itself for any significant food change in general. It will stop when the body reaches ketosis.

Most of the side effects of a keto diet are minor and temporary. But there are many controversies and some myths that scare people. Such as the misconception that your brain will stop working unless you eat a lot of carbohydrates. It's a myth that is due to a lack of understanding of how the body works in ketosis (changing the brain's fuel supply to ketones).

# Recipes

This section includes the recipes listed in the 14-day diet meal plan.

## 1. Scrambled eggs (one-pot meal)

Preparation time: 5 minutes

Cook time: 5 minutes

Ingredients for one serving:
Three eggs
½ shallot (or one small)
Some pickled peppers
One tomato
5 tbsp grated cheese
1½ tbsp butter or coconut oil
Salt
Pepper

Preparation:

i.   Finely chop the shallot, tomato, and pickled peppers.

ii.  In a bowl, break the eggs, beat them, and add the salt, pepper, and cheese.

iii. In a pan, put the butter and sauté the previously chopped vegetables for a few minutes. Then add the eggs and stir everything for a few minutes until you obtain the desired texture.

Nutritional value:
Per serving: cal: 378 kcal, net carbs: 1 g, fiber: 1 g, fat: 35 g, protein: 20 g.

## 2. Spinach and feta omelet (one-pot meal)
Total time: 10 mins

Ingredients for one serving:
2 tbsp onions, chopped
Four eggs
One pinch salt
2 oz feta cheese, crumbled
¼ cup spinach, chopped and cooked
Three tablespoons butter

Preparation:
i.    Break the four eggs into a small bowl, add the chopped onions and salt. Whisk the egg mixture thoroughly.
ii.   Melt three tablespoons of butter in a frying pan over medium heat and then add the egg mixture. Tip the pan to make sure the egg mixture covers the base of the pan.
iii.  Cook until the underside is lightly brown and then add the ¼ cup of spinach and the 2 oz crumbled feta cheese.
iv.   Use a spatula to fold the omelet into half.
v.    Lower the heat and cook until the inner part of the omelet is cooked (usually less than a minute).
vi.   Serve the omelet on a plate.

Nutritional value:
Per serving: cal: 870 kcal, net carbs: 5 g, fiber: 1 g, fat: 78 g, protein: 35 g.

## 3. Dairy-free latte (one-pot meal)

Preparation time: 5 minutes
Cooking time: 0 minute

Ingredients for two servings:
2 tbsp coconut oil
Two eggs
1½ cups boiling water
1 tsp ground ginger or pumpkin pie spice
One pinch vanilla extract

Preparation:
  i.   Put all ingredients in a blender and blend. Do this quickly to prevent the eggs from cooking in the boiling water! Drink right away.
  ii.  In case you simply want a plain latte or hot chocolate, use one tablespoon of cocoa or coffee in place of the spices.

Nutritional value:
Per serving: cal: 191 kcal, net carbs: 1 g, fiber: 0 g, fat: 18 g, protein: 6 g.

## 4. Keto fatty coffee (one-pot meal)

Total time: 5 minutes

Ingredients for one serving:
⅘ cups black coffee
¾ tbsp coconut oil
1½ tbsp sweet butter

Preparation:
  i.    In a shaker, mix the coffee with the butter and the coconut oil.
  ii.   Sweeten, if necessary, with a sweetener like stevia or erythritol.

Nutritional value:
Per serving: cal: 280 kcal, net carbs: 0 g, fiber: 0 g, fat: 31 g, protein: 0 g.

## 5. Avocado and pepper omelet (one-pot meal)
Total time: 6 minutes

Ingredients for one serving:
Two organic eggs
One avocado
½ minced onion
One chopped bell pepper
Salt
2 tsp of coconut oil

Preparation:

i.    Heat two teaspoons of coconut oil and add the eggs.

ii.   Add the onions and chopped peppers. Salt to taste.

iii.  Garnish your omelet with the avocado.

Nutritional value:
Per serving: cal: 539 kcal, net carbs: 3 g, fiber: 0 g, fat: 50 g, protein: 22 g.

# 6. Keto porridge of coconut and blueberries (one-pot meal)

Preparation time: 5 minutes
Cook time: 5 minutes

Ingredients for two servings:

For Porridge
¼ cup coconut flour
1 cup almond milk
¼ cup ground flaxseed
1 tsp vanilla extract
1 tsp cinnamon
One pinch salt
10 drops liquid stevia

For Toppings
2 oz blueberries
2 tbsp butter
1 oz. shaved coconut
2 tbsp pumpkin seeds

Preparation:
i.    On a low heat, heat a cup of almond milk in a pot.

ii.   Add coconut flour, flaxseed, cinnamon, and salt. Whisk to break up any clump.

iii.  Continue to heat until it bubbles slightly. Add in 1 tsp of vanilla extract and ten drops of liquid stevia.

iv.   Turn off the heat when you are satisfied with the thickness of the mixture. Add the butter, pumpkin seeds, blueberries, and shaved coconut as your toppings.

Nutritional value:
Per serving: cal: 412 kcal, net carbs: 7 g, fiber: 5 g, fat: 38 g, protein: 9 g.

## 7. Rolled smoked salmon, cream cheese and cucumber (one-pot meal)

Preparation: 10 min

Ingredients for one serving:
One slice of salmon
A small cucumber
2⅕ tbsp of fresh cheese
½ lemon
Dill
Salt and pepper

Preparation:
  i.  Rinse the cucumber, peel, and cut into small pieces.

  ii.  In a container, mix the cream cheese, cucumber pieces, juice of ½ lemon, dill, salt, and pepper to taste.

  iii.  Spread the mixture over the entire slice of salmon. Roll the slice and cut the roll horizontally to form small rolls.

Nutritional value:
Per serving: cal: 118 kcal, net carbs: 2 g, fat: 10 g, protein: 5 g.

# 8. Raspberry chia seed pudding

Preparation time: 10 minutes

Cook time: 10 minutes

Ingredients for two servings:
½ cup unsweetened coconut milk
¼ cup chia seeds
⅓ cup frozen raspberries
Cinnamon, vanilla extract or orange blossom, 1½ tbsp erythritol/stevia

Preparation:
i.   Mix the coconut milk and the chia seeds. Flavor with cinnamon, a few drops of vanilla extract, or orange blossom.
ii.  Place in the fridge for 2 hours.
iii. Meanwhile, thaw the raspberries.
iv.  Add the raspberries over the pudding, sprinkle with stevia/erythritol-type sweetener if needed, and enjoy.

Nutritional value:
Per serving: cal: 224 kcal, net carbs: 4 g, fiber: 8 g, fat: 18 g, protein: 6 g.

## 9. Peanut butter yogurt and cocoa powder (one-pot meal)
Total time: 5 minutes

Ingredients for two servings:
1 cup sugar-free yogurt
½ tbsp peanut butter
1 level tsp of cocoa powder
½ tsp stevia

Preparation:
  i.    Mix the yogurt with the peanut butter, cocoa powder, and stevia.

Nutritional value:
Per serving: cal: 430 kcal, net carbs: 5 g, fiber: 4 g, fat: 40 g, protein: 8 g.

## 10. Keto pancake (one-pot meal)

Preparation time: 5 minutes
Cook time: 10 minutes

Ingredients for three servings:
Two large eggs
One tbsp water
2 oz cream cheese, cubed
⅔ cup almond flour
One tsp baking powder
Two tsp vanilla extract
½ tsp cinnamon
½ tsp sweetleaf - stevia sweetener (or 2 tbsp regular sugar)
butter and syrup (sugar-free syrup for low carb option)

Preparation:
  i.    Add all ingredients except the butter and the syrup to the blender. Put the eggs, water, and cream cheese into the blender first. It helps to prevent anything from getting stuck to the bottom of the blender.
  ii.   Blend thoroughly until smooth. Let batter sit for two minutes.
  iii.  Apply medium heat to a non-stick skillet. Put 3-4 tablespoons of batter into a non-stick skillet for each pancake.
  iv.   Once it starts bubbling, flip. Continue to cook until both sides of the pancake turn brown. Do this until you have exhausted all the pancake batter.
  v.    Top the pancake with butter and syrup. Serve and enjoy.

Nutritional value:
Per serving: cal: 308 kcal, net carbs: 3 g, fiber: 2 g, fat: 28 g, protein: 10 g.

## 11. Chocolate chia pudding (one-pot meal)

Total time: 15 minutes

Ingredients for one serving:
¼ cup chia seeds
5 tbsp erythritol
¼ cup coconut milk
½ cup of water
1 tbsp raw cacao powder, unsweetened
5-10 drops stevia extract
½ tbsp raw cocoa nibs

Preparation:
i.    Mix the chia seeds, coconut milk, cacao powder, water, stevia, and erythritol. If you prefer a smoother texture, place it into a blender and pulse until smooth.
ii.   Let it sit for at least 10-15 minutes, ideally overnight in the fridge.
iii.  Top with cocoa nibs just before serving.

Nutritional value:
Per serving: cal: 330 kcal, net carbs: 6 g, fat: 27 g, protein: 10 g.

## 12. Keto sandwich

Total time: 20 minutes

Ingredients for two servings:
Four sausage patties
Two eggs
2 tbsp cream cheese
4 tbsp sharp cheddar
½ medium avocado, sliced
½-1 tsp sriracha (to taste)
Salt, pepper to taste

Preparation:
  i.    Heat a skillet over medium heat. Cook the four sausages in the skillet according to the instructions on the packaging and set aside.
  ii.   Put the cream cheese and sharp cheddar in a small bowl and microwave for about 20-30 seconds until melted.
  iii.  Mix the melted cheese with sriracha, and put aside.
  iv.   Break the two eggs into a bowl, whisk, add pepper and salt to taste. Mix well again and make the egg mixture into a small omelet.
  v.    Fill the omelet with the cheese sriracha mixture. Assemble the sandwich and spread the sliced avocado on top of the sandwich. Serve with the sausage and enjoy.

Nutritional value:
Per serving: cal: 601 kcal, net carbs: 4 g, fibre: 3 g, fat: 55 g, protein: 23 g.

## 13. Keto zucchini hash (one-pot meal)

Preparation time: 10 minutes
Cook time: 20 minutes

Ingredients for four servings:
Four small zucchini, grated and squeezed dry
Three tbsp coconut oil
One tbsp butter
⅓ cup grated parmesan cheese
One tsp chili powder, or more to taste
One tsp sea salt
One tsp cayenne pepper (optional)
Two eggs, beaten

Preparation:
    i.    Combine butter, zucchini, and coconut oil into a skillet and apply medium heat. Add the grated parmesan cheese, cayenne pepper, chili powder, and salt. Stir well.
    ii.    When the cheese melts, reduce the heat to low and add eggs. Stir again until thoroughly mixed. Return the heat to medium and cook until the edges of the hash are slightly brown. Stir and flip the hash occasionally while cooking.

Nutritional value:
Per serving: cal: 200 kcal, net carbs: 4 g, fat: 18 g, protein: 7 g.

## 14. Mushroom omelet (one-pot meal)

Preparation time: 10 minutes
Cook time: 20 minutes

Ingredients for one serving:
Three eggs
1 oz butter, for frying
1 oz shredded cheese
¼ yellow onion, chopped
Four large mushrooms, sliced
salt and pepper

Preparation:

i.  Break the three eggs into a small bowl, add pepper and salt to taste. Whisk the eggs properly. Heat a frying pan containing the butter over medium heat until the butter melts. Then add the chopped onions and the sliced mushrooms, stirring until tender. Pour the egg mixture into the pan.

ii. While cooking, sprinkle the shredded cheese on the little raw egg on the top before the omelet is thoroughly cooked.

iii. Ease the edges of the omelet with a spatula and fold it into half. Remove the frying pan from the heat when the lower side starts to turn to a golden brown. Serve the omelet on a plate.

Nutritional value:
Per serving: cal: 516 kcal, net carbs: 5 g, fibre: 1 g, fat: 45 g, protein: 26 g.

## 15. Keto cauliflower mac & cheese (one-pot meal)

Preparation time: 5 minutes
Cook time: 15 minutes

Ingredients for seven servings:
16 oz riced cauliflower
1 cup table cream
1 oz cream cheese, whipped
2 cups cheddar cheese, shredded
⅓ cup chives, minced
salt and pepper to taste

Preparation:
i. Preheat oven to 365 F.
ii. Heat an oiled skillet over medium heat.
iii. Place the riced cauliflower into the skillet and cook for about five minutes.
iv. Stir in cream, cream cheese, salt, pepper, and stir.
v. Add in 1 ½ cups of cheddar cheese and stir for about 2 minutes or until cheese is melted.
vi. Remove from heat and garnish with the remaining cup of cheddar cheese and chives.
vii. Broil until top is golden brown.

Nutritional value:
Per serving: cal: 197 kcal, net carbs: 3 g, fiber: 1 g, fat: 18 g, protein: 7 g.

## 16. Tuna with vegetables (one-pot meal)

Total time: 15 minutes

Ingredients for two servings:
½ cup celery finely chopped
One can tuna
2 tbsp honey mustard
½ cup carrot finely chopped
½ cup mayonnaise
1 cup red and yellow peppers finely chopped
2 tsp sweet relish
Salt

Preparation:

i.   Mix all the chopped vegetables in a bowl.

ii.  Add the tuna flakes and mix.

iii. Add mayonnaise, mustard, and sweet relish. Toss well.

iv.  Add salt to taste.

Nutritional value:
Per serving: cal: 339 kcal, net carbs: 4 g, fiber: 1 g, fat: 28 g, protein: 19 g.

## 17. Keto caprese omelet (one-pot meal)

Preparation time: 10 minutes
Cooking time: 10 minutes

Ingredients for two servings:
Six eggs
3 oz cherry tomatoes cut in equal parts or sliced tomatoes
2 tbsp olive oil
5 oz fresh mozzarella cheese, diced or sliced
1 tbsp chopped fresh or dried basil
salt and pepper

Preparation:

i.    Break the eggs into a bowl, add dark pepper and salt to your taste.

ii.    Whisk with a fork, add basil, and mix.

iii.    Heat oil in a pan, pour the tomatoes and fry for a couple of minutes.

iv.    Pour the egg batter on the tomatoes. Allow the batter to be slightly firm before including the mozzarella cheese.

v.    Reduce the heat and allow the omelet to set. Serve immediately and eat.

Nutritional value:
Per serving: cal: 534 kcal, net carbs: 4 g, fiber: 1 g, fat: 43 g, protein: 33 g.

## 18. Caesar keto salad (one-pot meal)

Total time: 10 minutes

Ingredients for four servings:

Salad

One head romaine lettuce

Four slices bacon cooked and crumbled

⅓ cup shredded parmesan cheese

Dressing
Three tbsp grated parmesan cheese
⅔ cup mayonnaise
¼ cup of sour cream
Two tsp fresh lemon juice
Two tsp worcestershire sauce
fresh black pepper
One clove garlic minced
½ tsp mustard powder
Two anchovy fillets or one tsp anchovy paste, minced

Preparation:

i.   Put the ingredients for the dressing in a small bowl and mix.

ii.  Place salad ingredients in a large bowl and top with a considerable quantity of the dressing. Mix properly and serve.

Nutritional value:
Per serving: cal: 461 kcal, net carbs: 4 g, fiber: 3 g, fat: 44 g, protein: 9 g.

## 19. Keto shrimp & artichoke plate (one-pot meal)

Total time: 15 minutes

Ingredients for two servings:
Four eggs
10 oz cooked and peeled shrimp
14 oz canned artichokes
Six sun-dried tomatoes in oil
½ cup mayonnaise
1½ oz baby spinach 4 tbsp
olive oil
salt and pepper

Preparation:
i.   Boil the eggs for about 4-8 minutes. Then cool the eggs in water for about 1-2 minutes to make it easy to peel the shell.
ii.  Place the eggs, artichokes, sun-dried tomatoes, mayonnaise, shrimp, and spinach on a plate.
iii. Sprinkle olive oil over the spinach and add pepper and salt to taste. Serve and enjoy.

Nutritional value:
Per serving: cal: 928 kcal, net carbs: 7 g, fiber: 7 g, fat: 80 g, protein: 36 g.

## 20. Smoked salmon-filled avocados (one-pot meal)

Total time: 10 minutes

Ingredients for one serving:
One medium avocado
3 oz smoked salmon
Four tbsp sour cream
Salt and pepper
One tbsp lemon juice

Preparation:
- i. Cut the avocado into two and put away the pit.
- ii. Put two tablespoons of the sour cream into the hollow parts of each half of avocado and add smoked salmon on top.
- iii. Add pepper and salt, and sprinkle the lemon juice on top.

Nutritional value:
Per serving: cal: 517 kcal, net carbs: 7 g, fat: 42 g, protein: 20 g.

## 21. Keto salami salad (one-pot meal)

Preparation time: 5 minutes
Cook time: 0 minute

Ingredients for two servings:
3½ oz salami slices
2 cups of spinach
One large avocado, diced
2 tbsp olive oil
One tsp balsamic vinegar

Preparation:

i.   Toss all the ingredients together.

Nutritional value:
Per serving: cal: 454 kcal, net carbs: 2 g, fibre: 8 g, fat: 42 g, protein: 9 g.

## 22. Spinach and bacon salad (one-pot meal)

Total time: 15 minutes

Ingredients for four servings:
8 oz spinach
Four large hard-boiled eggs
6 oz bacon
½ medium red onion, thinly sliced
½ cup mayonnaise
Salt and pepper

Preparation:
i. Put a pan over medium heat and cook the bacon in it until rendered and crispy. Chop into pieces when done and put aside.
ii. Slice the four large hard-boiled eggs.
iii. Place the rinsed spinach in a large bowl. Add mayonnaise, the remaining bacon fat, pepper, and salt to taste.
iv. Add the bacon, red onion, and sliced eggs into the salad and toss together. Serve immediately.

Nutritional value:
Per serving: cal: 509 kcal, net carbs: 3 g, fat: 46 g, protein: 20 g.

## 23. Keto BLT sandwich
Total time: 20 minutes

Ingredients for two servings:
Two slices of bacon
Two slices of iceberg lettuce
Two slices of tomato
½ avocado
Two tbsp mayonnaise
Four slices of keto bread
Salt and pepper

Preparation:
  i.    Place the slices of bacon in a frying pan, apply medium-high heat, and cook until crispy.
  ii.   Toast the four slices of keto bread in a toaster.
  iii.  Once done, layer the toasted bread with bacon, mayonnaise, lettuce, sliced avocado, and tomato.
  iv.   Season with pepper and salt. Serve!!!

Nutritional value:
Per serving: cal: 396 kcal, net carbs: 2 g, fibre: 6 g, fat: 37 g, protein: 10 g.

## 24. Keto Italian plate (one-pot meal)

Preparation time: 5 minutes
Cooking time: 0 minute

Ingredients for two servings:
7 oz fresh mozzarella cheese
⅓ cup olive oil
Two tomatoes
Ten green olives
7 oz prosciutto, sliced
salt and pepper

Preparation:
  i.   Put the prosciutto, olives, tomatoes, and cheese on a plate.
       Then, add pepper and salt to taste. Serve with olive oil.

Nutritional value:
Per serving: cal: 822 kcal, net carbs: 8 g, fiber: 3 g, fat: 69 g,
protein: 40 g.

## 25. Keto crustless pizza

Preparation time: 5 minutes
Cook time: 10 minutes

Ingredients for one serving:
½ green bell pepper cut in slices
1 oz turkey ham cut in small squares
1 tbsp red onion cut in slices
2 tbsp Rao's Pizza Sauce (or tomato paste)
½ tbsp olive oil
1 oz mozzarella cheese grated

Preparation:
  i.   Preheat a frying pan and then pour the oil in. Fry the ham for 3 minutes. Optionally, use any meat of your choice instead of ham. Put aside.
  ii.  Set the bell pepper on the base of a microwave-safe bowl and layer with the onion, ham, and tomato paste.
  iii. Top with mozzarella.
  iv.  Microwave for 3 minutes and let the cheese melt. As an alternative, bake for 10 minutes in the oven preheated at 370 F. Remember to use an oven-safe pan for this.
  v.   Take out from the microwave (or oven) and enjoy it.

Nutritional value:
Per serving: cal: 239 kcal, net carbs: 5 g, fibre: 1 g, fat: 18 g, protein: 13 g.

## 26. Chicken no-noodle soup (one-pot meal)

Preparation time: 10 minutes
Cook time: 20 minutes

Ingredients for four servings:
One tsp olive oil
One medium onion, diced
Four carrots, sliced
Four stalks celery, diced
½ lb boneless skinless chicken breast
32 oz reduced sodium chicken broth
Four sprigs thyme
Two bay leaves
2 cups cooked spaghetti squash
salt and pepper to taste

Preparation:
i.   Apply heat to a large soup pot containing olive oil and saute onion, carrots, and celery until softened.
ii.  Add chicken breast, chicken broth, thyme, bay leaves, salt, and pepper. Bring to a boil until chicken is cooked.
iii. Remove chicken from the pot and shred. Add it back to the pot after shredding.
iv.  Stir it in spaghetti squash and serve.

Nutritional value:
Per serving: cal: 507 kcal, net carbs: 4 g, fibre: 1 g, fat: 40 g, protein: 31 g.

## 27. Keto frittata with avocado and queso (one-pot meal)

Preparation time: 10 minutes
Cook time: 15 minutes

Ingredients for six servings:
Eight eggs
One teaspoon taco seasoning
¼ cup heavy cream
½ cup shredded monterey jack cheese
4 oz cotija cheese
½ cup cherry tomatoes, halved
4 oz can diced green chiles
¼ cup sliced green onion
One avocado, cut into slices
Four slices of bacon

Preparation:
i. Preheat the oven to 400 F. Also, crack the eggs into a large bowl, add cream and taco spices, and whisk all together.
ii. Cook bacon in a 10.5″ cast-iron skillet over medium-high heat until crispy. Remove the bacon from the skillet, chop, and drain off all but two tablespoons of the fat.
iii. Add the egg mixture, green chiles, onion, and jack cheese to the skillet. Make the toppings with cherry tomatoes halves, bacon crumbles, crumbled cojita, and avocado slices.
iv. Bake for about 12-15 minutes in the oven at 400 F. Slice and serve.

Nutritional value:
Per serving: cal: 322 kcal, net carbs: 4 g, fibre: 3 g, fat: 26 g, protein: 18 g.

## 28. Keto smoked mackerel salad

Preparation time: 10 minutes
Cook time: 20 minutes

Ingredients for one serving:
1 small tomato
1 large egg
1 oz red onion
2 fillet smoked mackerel
¼ tsp salt
2 tbsp olive oil
2½ oz avocado
⅓ tbsp black pepper
1 tbsp pumpkin seeds
1 tbsp fresh lime juice
2 cup baby spinach

Preparation:
i.    To a frying pan containing a tablespoon of olive oil, apply a medium-high heat. Add the mackerel and fry for about 3-4 minutes until golden. Flip the mackerel and cook for another 1-2 minutes or until the fish is thoroughly cooked. Flake the fish into bite-sizes and put aside.
ii.   Add the spinach to a salad bowl. Dice the tomato, avocado, and onion. Add the diced constituents to the bowl containing the spinach and toss well to combine.
iii.  Cook the egg and peel off the shell when the egg is chilled. Make the dressing by mixing all the ingredients - flaked mackerel, lime juice, remaining olive oil, salt, and pepper. Toss well to combine.
iv.   Add sliced eggs on the dressing. Scatter with the pumpkin seeds to serve.

Nutritional value:
Per serving: cal: 441 kcal, net carbs: 4 g, fibre: 4 g, fat: 39 g, protein: 13 g.

## 29. Keto carbonara

Preparation time: 5 minutes
Cooking time: 10 minutes

Ingredients for two servings:
2 cups zucchini spaghetti
7 oz smoked bacon cubes
One egg
One egg yolk
1⅔ oz parmesan cheese
Black pepper
Salt

Preparation:
  i.    Mix the egg, the egg yolk, the cheese, and black pepper.
  ii.   Spiralize the zucchini and make the spaghetti.
  iii.  Fry the bacon starting in a cold pan to render the fat.
  iv.   Once the fat has rendered and the bacon is crisp, remove excess oil, if any.
  v.    Add the zucchini, add some salt, and cook till tender.
  vi.   Turn off the heat and pour in the egg mixture and mix through the spaghetti till everything is well coated.
  vii.  Sprinkle some freshly grated parmesan on top.

Nutritional value:
Per serving: cal: 601 kcal, net carbs: 2 g, fiber: 3 g, fat: 54 g, protein: 24 g.

## 30. Shrimp avocado cucumber salad

Preparation time: 10 minutes
Cooking time: 5 minutes

Ingredients for four servings:

For the Shrimp
26-39 uncooked extra-large shrimp (peeled and deveined)
One tbsp butter
One tbsp olive oil
Salt and black pepper

For the Salad
1½ cups of chopped cucumber
½ cup of chopped red onions
1 cup chopped red bell pepper
Two medium avocado — peeled, pitted and chopped
One tbsp parsley — chopped
Two tbsp lemon juice
Four tbsp olive oil
Salt and black pepper

Preparation:
  i.    Pat the dry shrimps with a paper towel.
  ii.   Apply medium-high heat to a skillet containing the olive oil and butter. Add shrimps, pepper, and salt
  iii.  Cook until done or for about 1-2 minutes.
  iv.   In a large salad bowl, add cucumber, red onions, bell pepper, avocado, parsley, and shrimp.
  v.    Pour the lemon juice, olive oil, black pepper, and salt to taste into a small bowl. Whisk until combined.
  vi.   Pour the seasoning over the salad.
  vii.  Toss to combine and enjoy.

Nutritional value:
Per serving: cal: 314 kcal, net carbs: 5 g, fiber: 6 g, fat: 24 g, protein: 18 g.

## 31. Pesto chicken and veggies (one-pot meal)
Preparation time: 10 minutes
Cooking time: 20 minutes

Ingredients for four servings:
Two tbsp olive oil
⅓ cup of chopped sun-dried tomatoes drained of oil
¼ cup basil pesto
1 lb skinless and boneless chicken thighs, sliced
1 lb asparagus ends trimmed, cut in half, if large
1 cup cherry tomatoes, halved
Salt

Preparation:
i.   Heat a large skillet on medium heat. Add two tablespoons of olive oil, sliced chicken thighs, and season chicken generously with salt. Also, add half of the chopped sun-dried tomatoes to the skillet and cook for about 5-10 minutes. Turn the sides until the chicken is thoroughly cooked. Remove the chicken and sun-dried tomatoes from the skillet, and leave the oil in n the skillet.
ii.  Add asparagus (ends trimmed) to the skillet, add the remaining half of the sun-dried tomatoes, season generously with salt, and cook for about 5-10 minutes until the asparagus is cooked. Remove the asparagus and serve on a plate.
iii. Return the chicken to the skillet, add pesto, and stir to coat on low-medium heat until chicken is reheated, for one or two minutes. Remove the skillet from heat. Add halved cherry tomatoes to the skillet and mix all together. Add chicken and tomatoes to the serving plate with asparagus.

Nutritional value:
Per serving: cal: 423 kcal, net carbs: 5 g, fiber: 4 g, fat: 32 g, protein: 23 g.

## 32. Salmon with walnut-avocado guacamole
Total time: 20 minutes

Ingredients for four servings:
4 (6 oz) skin-on salmon fillets
1 tsp kosher salt, divided
½ teaspoon black pepper, divided
⅓ cup toasted walnuts, divided
4 tbsp extra-virgin olive oil, divided
1½ tablespoons fresh lime juice
1 peeled ripe avocado
5 cups baby arugula
¾ cup thinly sliced radishes

Preparation:
  i.   Heat a grill pan over medium-high heat.
  ii.  Sprinkle the salmon with ¼ tsp salt and ¼ tsp pepper; use the cooking spray to coat the grill pan. Place the salmon fillets, with the part containing the skin-side down, and cook for 5 minutes. Turn and cook for about 3 minutes until done.
  iii. Place ½ tsp salt, remaining ¼ tsp pepper, ¼ cup walnuts, 2½ tbsp extra-virgin olive oil, 1½ tbsp lime juice, and avocado in a food processor. Pulse until almost smooth.
  iv.  Place the remaining ¼ tsp salt, arugula, and radishes in a large bowl. Add the remaining 1½ tsp extra-virgin olive oil; toss. Divide the salad among four plates. Make toppings with guacamole and salmon. Chop the remaining walnuts, and sprinkle on top.

Nutritional value:
Per serving: cal: 461 kcal, net carbs: 2 g, fibre:  4g, fat: 33 g, protein: 37 g.

## 33. Zoodles with creamy salmon sauce

Preparation time: 15 minutes
Cooking time: 15 minutes

Ingredients for four servings:
2 lbs zucchini
2 tbsp olive oil
salt and pepper
1 cup heavy whipping cream
4 oz. cream cheese
¼ cup chopped fresh basil or fresh cilantro
One lime, juiced
1 lb smoked salmon

Preparation:
  i.   Rinse and cut the zucchini into thin, pasta-like strips using a mandolin
  ii.  Place the zucchini and salt in a colander, and mix properly to coat the strips with the salt. Put it aside for about 5-10 minutes and then press to discard excess liquid.
  iii. Mix the cream, lime juice, and cream cheese in a small saucepan. While stirring, cook for a few minutes until it simmers.
  iv.  Reduce the heat and add herbs together with the smoked salmon. Cut the salmon into thin strips and season with pepper and salt.
  v.   Add oil to a frying pan and put over medium-high heat. Add zucchini spirals and fry for about 1-2 minutes. Season with pepper and salt. Serve immediately with the sauce.

Nutritional value:
Per serving: cal: 537 kcal, net carbs: 9 g, fiber: 3 g, fat: 44 g, protein: 27 g.

## 34. Spicy kimchi ahi poke

Total time: 10 minutes

Ingredients for four servings:
1 lb sushi-grade ahi tuna, diced
sesame seeds
One ripe avocado, diced
1 tbsp soy sauce
½ tsp sesame oil
2 tbsp sriracha
½ cup kimchi
¼ cup mayonnaise
chopped green onion

Preparation:
   i.   Add the diced ahi tuna, mayonnaise, soy sauce, sesame oil, and sriracha to a mixing bowl and toss to combine.
   ii.  Also, add diced avocado and kimchi to the bowl and gently combine.
   iii. Serve it on top of traditional rice, salad greens, or cauli rice, or traditional rice and sprinkle the sesame seeds and chopped green onion on top.

Nutritional value
Per serving: cal: 299 kcal, net carbs: 3 g, fiber: 1 g, fat: 18 g, protein: 5 g.

## 35. Ketogenic pizza

Preparation time: 5 minutes
Cooking time: 25 minutes

Ingredients for two servings:
  6 oz. shredded mozzarella cheese
  Four eggs

Toppings
  1 tsp oregano, dried
  olives (optional)
  3 tbsp unsweetened tomato sauce
  5 oz shredded mozzarella cheese
  1½ oz thinly sliced pepperoni

Dressing
  4 tbsp olive oil
  2 oz vegetable greens
  salt and black pepper (ground)

Preparation:
  i.    Start by heating the oven to about 400 F. Line a pizza pan with parchment paper.
  ii.   Start by preparing the crust. Break the four eggs and add 6 oz shredded mozzarella cheese into the same bowl. Mix adequately.
  iii.  Spread the egg batter and cheese with a spatula on the lined pizza pan. Frame it into two circles or a big rectangle. Bake pizza for about 12 minutes until the crust turns golden. Take it out of the oven and let it cool for about two minutes.
  iv.   Raise the temperature of the oven to about 450 F.
  v.    Spread the unsweetened tomato sauce and sprinkle the dried oregano on the crust. Top with 5 oz mozzarella cheese, olives, and pepperoni.
  vi.   Bake the pizza again for about 8 minutes, until golden brown.
  vii.  Make the dressing by mixing all the ingredients – olive oil, vegetable greens, salt, and black pepper. Toss well to combine. Serve!!!

Nutritional value:
Per serving: cal: 1043 kcal, net carbs: 5 g, fiber: 1 g, fat: 90 g, protein: 53 g.

## 36. Keto fried chicken and broccoli (one-pot meal)

Preparation time: 5 minutes
Cooking time: 15 minutes

Ingredients for two servings:
9 oz broccoli
3½ oz butter
10 oz boneless, skinless, chicken thighs
Salt and pepper, to taste

Preparation:
i. Rinse the broccoli (including the stems) and cut it into smaller bite-sizes.
ii. Heat a pan containing half of the butter over medium-high heat.
iii. Season the chicken with pepper and salt to taste. Once the pan is hot, and the butter is melted, add the seasoned chicken to the pan and cook until golden brown, each side for about 5 minutes.
iv. Add the bite-sized broccoli and the remaining butter to the pan and saute for a few more minutes. Add additional salt if there is any need.
v. Serve it with all of the pan drippings, using the broccoli to soak up the pan drippings.

Nutritional value:
Per serving: cal: 603 kcal, net carbs: 5 g, fat: 54 g, protein: 28 g.

## 37. Eggs with salmon and spinach (one-pot meal)

Preparation time: 5 minutes
Cooking time: 0 minute

Ingredients for 3 servings:
1 lb frozen leeks with cream
14 oz pink salmon
Four eggs
One tsp of spinach
½ red pepper

Preparation:
i.    Preheat the oven to 347 F.
ii.   Mix all the ingredients.
iii.  Pour into muffin tins, almost to the edge.
iv.   Bake for about 15 minutes.

Nutritional value:
Per serving: cal: 554 kcal, net carbs: 2 g, fibre: 0g, fat: 41 g, protein: 32 g.

## 38. Cabbage and bacon keto

Preparation time: 5 minutes
Cooking time: 15 minutes

Ingredients for two servings:
6 oz bacon
16 oz green cabbage
Two tbsp butter
Salt and pepper, to taste

Preparation:
i.    Cut the green cabbage and bacon into small bite-sizes.
ii.   Put the bacon in a pan and cook over medium heat until the bacon is rendered and crispy.
iii.  Add the green cabbage and butter to the pan, and season with pepper and salt to taste. Fry the green cabbage until slightly soft and golden.
iv.   Serve it with the pan drippings.

Nutritional value:
Per serving: cal: 612 kcal, net carbs: 7 g, fat: 51 g, protein: 25 g.

## 39. Keto apple Dijon pork chops

Preparation time: 5 minutes
Cook time: 10 minutes

Ingredients for two servings:
Two pork chops
6 tbsp of ghee
2 tbsp of applesauce
2 tbsp of ghee
2 tbsp of Dijon mustard
Salt and pepper, to taste

Preparation:
   i.   Put four tablespoons of ghee in a large pan and melt over medium heat.
   ii.   Add the pork chops to the pan. Use tongs to position the pork chops on its side so that the fat cooks in the ghee first, to render the fat a bit. Again, lay the pork chops flat when the fat is a bit crispy and browned.
   iii.   Cook each side for about 3-4 minutes. Read the internal temperature of the pork and ensure it reaches 145 F. You can choose to extend the cooking for much longer to your satisfaction.
   iv.   Meanwhile, mix the apple sauce, the remaining two tablespoons of ghee, and Dijon mustard.
   v.   Serve the pork chops with the sauce. Season with pepper and salt to taste.

Nutritional value:
Per serving: cal: 560 kcal, net carbs: 2 g, fibre: 4 g, fat: 49 g, protein: 34 g.

# 40. Mexican cauliflower rice skillet (one-pot meal)

Preparation time: 5 minutes
Cook time: 20 minutes

Ingredients for six servings:
1 lb ground beef
¼ medium onion diced
½ red pepper diced
3 tbsp taco seasoning
1 cup diced tomatoes
12 oz cauliflower rice fresh or frozen
½ cup chicken broth
1½ cups shredded cheddar cheese

Preparation:
i.   Place the ground beef in a large skillet and cook over medium heat. Add onion and pepper and continue to cook until it is brown. Add the taco seasoning and stir.
ii.  Add the tomatoes and cauliflower rice and stir to combine. Stir in the broth and allow it to simmer. Reduce the heat to medium-low and cook until the cauliflower rice begins to soften (8 to 10 minutes for frozen).
iii. Sprinkle the shredded cheddar cheese in the skillet and cover. Allow cooking for about 3 or 4 minutes until the cheese melts. Remove from heat and top with your favorite toppings like sour cream, avocado, and chopped cilantro.

Nutritional value:
Per serving: cal: 352 kcal, net carbs: 5 g, fibre: 4 g, fat: 22 g, protein: 29 g.

## 41. Salmon with asparagus & quick blender hollandaise
Total time: 15 minutes

Ingredients for two servings:
1 tbsp avocado oil
8½ oz small wild salmon fillets
8½ oz small bunch asparagus
Two large egg yolks
6 tbsp unsalted butter or ghee, melted
1 tbsp fresh lemon juice
pinch of cayenne pepper
water (if too thick)
salt and pepper, to taste

Preparation:
i.    Place one tablespoon of avocado oil in a cast-iron skillet and apply a medium-high heat. Season the salmon with pepper and salt and place skin side down in the skillet. Sear 4-5 minutes until the salmon easily releases from the bottom of the pan.
ii.   Turn and continue to sear for another 4-5 minutes until it releases again.
iii.  Turn again and add the asparagus to the skillet. Cook for about 3-4 minutes, tossing a few times, so that each stalk gets seared. Set aside.
iv.   To prepare the hollandaise sauce, heat the butter over medium heat until melted and bubbling. Remove the pan from the heat.
v.    Put the egg yolks, lemon juice, and cayenne in a blender and blend for about 30 seconds until the egg yolks are broken. Stream in the bubbling butter slowly and steadily while the blender runs. The sauce should thicken. Add some water and blend if it is too thick.
vi.   Season with salt, pepper, and cayenne pepper and pour over the salmon and asparagus.
vii.  Serve it on a plate or store it in the refrigerator for a day. Hollandaise is best served fresh.

Nutritional value:
Per serving: cal: 631 kcal, net carbs: 3 g, fat: 54 g, protein: 30 g.

## 42. Oven baked trout with mustard glaze (one-pot meal)
Total time: 30 minutes

Ingredients for two servings:
Six tbsp apple cider vinegar
Two tbsp Dijon or yellow mustard
Three tbsp avocado oil or melted ghee
Two trout fillets (about 6 ounces each)
One tbsp raw organic honey

Preparation:
i. Preheat oven to 420 F.
ii. Mix the vinegar, mustard, and the avocado oil or melted ghee in a bowl. Whisk together until thoroughly combined with no clumps.
iii. Place trout fillets in a bag or shallow dish and pour about ⅔ of the marinade over the fish. Reserve about ⅓ of the mixture for later.
iv. Marinate for about 15 minutes.
v. Place fish fillets on a baking dish and bake for 12 minutes.
vi. To serve, add the honey to the remaining marinade mixture and pour over the cooked fish.

Nutritional value:
Per serving: cal: 449 kcal, net carbs: 8 g, fat: 42 g, protein: 34 g.

# Food shopping & pantry list

Here is my ideal shopping list, which will be very useful for you to lose weight. Sometimes it is difficult to purchase because the supermarket is full of temptations. Buying the healthiest foods possible and identifying those with fewer calories, but which keep you full and adequately supplied with nutrients, is a significant commitment, that only those who go shopping every day and care about choosing healthy and light food can understand.

So, I took a lot of time to research on the nutrient profiles of the best foods to eat, which are not only good for our body but also help us lose weight. Below you'll find your go-to keto grocery list filled with keto-friendly foods:

- Dairy Products/Eggs:
  - Eggs
  - Unsweetened yogurt
  - Cottage cheese
  - Cream cheese
  - Mayonnaise
  - Heavy whipping cream
  - Greek yogurt
  - Butter (grass-fed preferred)

- Nuts & Seeds:
  - Walnuts
  - Hazelnuts

- Pecans
- Almonds
- Chia seeds
- Pumpkin seeds
- Flaxseeds
- Sunflower seeds
- Macadamias

- Fats:
  - MCT oil
  - Olive oil
  - Lard
  - Avocado oil
  - Sesame oil
  - Coconut oil
  - Ghee
  - Coconut butter
  - Peanut butter
  - Canola oil
  - Extra virgin olive oil
- Meats:
  - Ground beef
  - Chicken
  - Ham
  - Turkey

- o Pepperoni
- o Salmon
- o Pork
- o Fish and Shellfish
- o Bacon
- o Sausages

- Vegetables:
  - o Broccoli
  - o Spinach
  - o Red Onions
  - o Cauliflower
  - o Artichokes
  - o Cabbage
  - o Mushrooms
  - o Celery
  - o Kale
  - o Garlic
  - o Cucumber
  - o Pepper
  - o Zucchini
- Fruits:
  - o Lemon
  - o Avocado
  - o Berries

- o Lime
- o Watermelon
- Pantry items:
  - o Bone broth
  - o Stevia or Erythritol
  - o Salad dressings (low carb varieties)
  - o Baking cocoa powder
  - o Cinnamon
  - o Pesto
  - o Turmeric
  - o Paprika
  - o Thyme
  - o Beef broth
  - o Chicken broth
  - o Salad dressing
  - o Ranch dressing
  - o Caesar dressing
  - o Dijon mustard
  - o Cilantro
  - o Curry powder

# Conclusion

The keto diet, known as a low-carb and high-fat diet, offers various health benefits, which include weight loss. While the exact mode of action of achieving weight loss is still under investigation, it most likely results from a calorie deficit, reduction in hunger levels, and water weight loss. If you stick with it, the benefits of a ketogenic diet are awe-inspiring.

Keto supplements also play a substantial role in helping to reduce hunger and to reach ketosis more rapidly; however, they should not be used to promote weight loss. A ketogenic diet may be an option for some people who have had difficulty losing weight with other methods. Therefore, keto diet starters should consult a physician or a dietitian to monitor any biochemical changes after starting the regimen and to create a meal plan that suits one's existing health conditions helping to prevent nutritional deficiencies or other health complications.

Made in the USA
Coppell, TX
03 December 2024

41726840R00052